ENHANCE YOUR BRAIN

Strategies for Improving Mental Health and Well-being

James Stowers

Table of contents

Introduction

The Importance of Brain Health

Brain health is a key part of general health and well-being, playing a critical role in everything from our thoughts and emotions to our capacity to move and do daily chores. Despite its significance, brain health is frequently ignored and not given the attention it needs. This is unfortunate since there are numerous strategies to improve and maintain brain health, leading to a higher quality of life, increased cognitive ability, and lower risk of cognitive decline and brain illnesses.

The brain is a complex organ that is responsible for a vast variety of processes, including perception, thinking, emotion, movement, and memory. It is also the heart of our awareness and the wellspring of our unique personality and identity. Given its significance, it is crucial that we take care of our brains and preserve their health and well-being.

One of the most efficient methods to preserve brain health is regular physical activity. Exercise has been demonstrated to have a major beneficial influence on brain health, boosting cognitive performance, lowering the risk of cognitive decline and brain diseases, and promoting brain plasticity. Exercise also boosts blood flow to the brain, providing it with the essential oxygen and nutrients to perform at its optimum.

In addition to physical activity, good sleep is also crucial for brain health. Sleep is crucial for the consolidation of memories and the healing and restoration of the brain and body. During sleep, the brain clears off waste and poisons, enabling it to operate properly while awake. Poor sleep, on the other hand, may contribute to cognitive decline, memory issues, and an increased risk of brain illnesses.

Nutrition also plays a key influence on brain health. A diet that is rich in vital nutrients, such as omega-3 fatty acids, antioxidants, and vitamins B and D, may have a substantial influence on brain function, boosting memory and cognitive capacity, and lowering the risk of cognitive decline and brain illnesses.

Stimulation and learning are also vital for preserving brain function. Engaging in activities that challenge the brain, such as reading, solving puzzles, and learning a new skill, may assist to increase cognitive ability and sustain brain function. By exposing the brain to new experiences and knowledge, we can maintain it active and healthy, lowering the risk of cognitive decline.

Stress management is particularly crucial for brain health, since prolonged stress may have a harmful impact on the brain and contribute to cognitive decline. Practicing stress-reducing activities, such as meditation, deep breathing, and exercise, may assist to lessen the detrimental effects of stress and preserve brain health.

Finally, social engagement is critical for brain health, since social contact and relationships play a significant role in our general well-being and cognitive performance. Studies have revealed that social isolation and loneliness may have a major detrimental influence on brain health, leading to cognitive decline and an increased risk of brain illnesses. By preserving social ties and interactions, we may increase our brain health and lower the risk of cognitive decline.

In conclusion, brain health is vital for general health and well-being, and there are various strategies to maintain and enhance it. From exercise and sleep to nutrition, stimulation and learning, stress management, and social engagement, many factors can impact brain health, and by paying attention to these, we can reduce the risk of cognitive decline and brain disorders, leading to a better quality of life and enhanced cognitive abilities.

Brain health is a critical part of general health and well-being since the brain governs and coordinates all the processes of the body. A healthy brain is necessary for sustaining cognitive functions, such as memory, learning, and problem-solving, as well as emotional stability, mental clarity, and the capacity to make choices and accomplish daily activities.

One of the major components in preserving brain health is participating in regular physical activity. Exercise has been demonstrated to have a favorable influence on brain function by improving blood flow to the brain and giving it the essential oxygen and nutrients to perform at its optimum. Exercise also helps to decrease stress and anxiety, both of which may have a bad influence on brain function.

Adequate sleep is also crucial for brain health, as it gives the brain the time it needs to consolidate memories, repair and rejuvenate itself, and clear away waste and toxins. Sleep deprivation may lead to cognitive decline, memory issues, and an increased risk of brain illnesses, such as depression and Alzheimer's disease.

Nutrition is another crucial aspect of brain health, as a diet that is rich in necessary nutrients may boost cognitive skills, increase memory, and minimize the risk of cognitive decline and brain illnesses. Nutrients such as omega-3 fatty acids, antioxidants, and vitamins B and D are especially essential for brain health since they serve to protect the brain from harm and maintain its function.

Stimulation and learning are also vital for sustaining brain health since they serve to keep the brain active and engaged. Engaging in activities that challenge the brain, such as reading, solving puzzles, and learning a new skill, may assist to increase cognitive ability and sustain brain function. By exposing the brain to new experiences and knowledge, we can maintain it active and healthy, lowering the risk of cognitive decline.

Stress management is also critical for brain health, since prolonged stress may have a negative impact on the brain and contribute to cognitive impairment. Practicing stress-reducing activities, such as meditation, deep breathing, and exercise, may assist to lessen the detrimental effects of stress and preserve brain health.

Finally, social engagement is critical for brain health, since social contact and relationships play a significant role in our general well-being and cognitive performance. Studies have revealed that social isolation and loneliness may have a major detrimental influence on brain health, leading to cognitive decline and an increased risk of brain illnesses. By preserving social ties and interactions, we may increase our brain health and lower the risk of cognitive decline.

In conclusion, brain health is vital for general health and well-being, and there are various strategies to maintain and enhance it. From exercise and sleep to nutrition, stimulation and learning, stress management, and social engagement, many factors can impact brain health, and by paying attention to these, we can reduce the risk of cognitive decline and brain disorders, leading to a better quality of life and enhanced cognitive abilities. By taking care of our brains, we can guarantee that we have the cognitive and emotional stability, mental clarity, and capacity to make choices that we need to lead satisfying and productive lives.

The concept of Neuroplasticity

The ability of the brain to adapt and change in response to new experiences, learning, and environmental cues is known as neuroplasticity. We can learn new abilities, create new memories, and adjust to new settings because of this essential component of how the brain works.

Our knowledge of the brain and its capacity for change has been completely transformed by the concept of neuroplasticity, a relatively new advancement in the field of neuroscience. It used to be thought that the brain was a fixed structure with distinct regions assigned to different functions and that changes in the brain were minimal and mostly happened during early development.

The brain is significantly more elastic and adaptable than previously believed, and changes can take place throughout life, according to a current study.

The development of new brain connections, or synapses, between neurons in response to learning, new experiences, and environmental stimuli is one of the main mechanisms of neuroplasticity. Synaptic plasticity is a process that enables the brain to adjust and transform in response to novel experiences. For instance, new brain connections are created as a result of new experiences and learning when we learn a new ability, like playing an instrument. This allows us to gradually improve and hone our talents.

The brain's capacity to reorganize itself in response to trauma or illness is a crucial feature of neuroplasticity. We can recover from damage or sickness and maintain cognitive and motor functions because of a mechanism known as adaptive plasticity that enables the brain to compensate for the loss of function in one area by rerouting impulses to other parts of the brain. For instance, the brain can reorganize itself after a stroke to compensate for the loss of function in one area, restoring part of the person's talents and a measure of their independence.

The fact that our thoughts, attitudes, and behaviors can have an impact on neuroplasticity is one of its most remarkable features. Studies have demonstrated, for instance, that while stress and anxiety can negatively affect neuroplasticity and cause changes in the brain that might result in cognitive loss, positive thinking, and self-reflection can boost neuroplasticity and cause changes in the brain.

Our capacity to create and retrieve memories is significantly influenced by neuroplasticity. The creation of new synaptic connections, the strengthening of preexisting connections, and the restructuring of neuronal circuits all play important roles in the complex processes of memory formation and recall. The capacity of the brain to adapt to new experiences is crucial for memory formation and recall, and studies have shown that challenging mental tasks like picking up a new skill or playing an instrument can promote neuroplasticity and improve memory creation and recall.

Education, therapy, and health are just a few of the areas of our life where the idea of neuroplasticity has broad ramifications. Understanding neuroplasticity has sparked the development of novel learning strategies in education, such as brain-based learning, which makes use of the brain's capacity for change and adaptation to enhance learning and enhance results. By focusing on the underlying mechanisms of neuroplasticity to speed healing and improve results, new ways to treat brain illnesses like traumatic brain injury and depression have been developed as a result of research on neuroplasticity. By focusing on neuroplasticity's mechanisms to speed recovery and increase results, new treatments for neurological diseases like stroke have been made possible because of advances in medical science.

In summary, neuroplasticity is an essential feature of the brain.

The term "neuroplasticity" describes the brain's capacity to alter, adapt, and restructure itself in response to fresh experiences, new knowledge, and outside stimuli. We are able to learn new skills, create new memories, and adjust to new circumstances because of the brain's capacity for change. Formerly believed to only occur during early development, current studies have revealed that the brain may change and adapt throughout life.

The development of new brain connections, or synapses, between neurons in response to learning, new experiences, and environmental stimuli is one of the main mechanisms of neuroplasticity. The brain may adapt and alter in response to new knowledge thanks to a process known as synaptic plasticity. As an illustration, when you learn to play an instrument, new brain connections are created in response to the learning and experience, enabling you to hone and develop your talents over time.

The brain's capacity to reorganize itself in response to trauma or illness is a crucial feature of neuroplasticity. People can recover from injury or illness and maintain cognitively and motor functions thanks to a mechanism known as adaptive plasticity that enables the brain to compensate for the loss of function in one area by rerouting impulses to other parts of the brain. For instance, the brain can rewire itself after a stroke to make up for the lost function, enabling the affected individual to regain a part of their talents and their independence.

Neuroplasticity is influenced by our thoughts, attitudes, and behaviors in addition to our experiences and surroundings. For instance, research has shown that while stress and worry can have the reverse impact and cause changes in the brain that can end in cognitive loss, positive thinking and self-reflection can promote neuroplasticity and lead to changes in the brain.

Neuroplasticity is also intimately linked to memory formation and recall. New synaptic connections are formed, existing connections are strengthened, and neuronal circuits are reorganized during memory formation and recall. Learning a new skill or playing an instrument are examples of mentally taxing activities that have been demonstrated to boost neuroplasticity and enhance memory development and recall.

The idea of neuroplasticity has significant effects on treatment, medicine, and education. Understanding neuroplasticity has sparked the development of novel learning strategies in education, such as brain-based learning, which makes use of the brain's capacity for change to improve learning and outcomes. By focusing on neuroplasticity's underlying mechanisms to enhance recovery and outcomes, new therapeutic strategies have been developed in therapy to treat brain illnesses like depression and traumatic brain injury. By focusing on neuroplasticity's mechanisms to speed recovery and increase results, new treatments for neurological diseases like stroke have been made possible because of advances in medical science.

In conclusion, neuroplasticity is an essential component of brain function that enables learning, adaptation, and recovery from illness or injury. Our ability to build new memories, pick up new abilities, and recover from illness or injury is all made possible by the brain's capacity to adapt to new experiences and external stimuli. Learning about neuroplasticity has significant ramifications for therapy, health, and education. It has also sparked the creation of fresh methods for treating brain problems and enhancing learning.

Understanding Brain Function

The human brain is the control center for our ideas, emotions, actions, and movements. It is an extraordinarily complex and clever organ that enables us to experience the world around us, think, learn, and create. Despite its complexity, scientists have been able to make enormous progress in understanding how the brain functions, including how neurons connect with one another, how memories are generated, and how humans absorb information.

The brain is made of billions of neurons, or nerve cells, which interact with each other via electrical and chemical impulses. Neurons are joined by specialized structures called synapses, which enable them to relay impulses to one another. When one neuron gets a signal, it passes it on to the next cell via the production of substances called neurotransmitters. This mechanism is known as synaptic transmission, and it allows neurons to connect with one another, enabling us to interpret and react to information from our surroundings.

One of the major jobs of the brain is to process and react to sensory information from the environment. This process begins with the sensory receptors, such as the eyes and hearing, which detect and transform sensory information into electrical impulses that are delivered to the brain. The brain then interprets this information and develops a reaction, such as a muscular movement or a behavioral change.

Memory formation and recall are also crucial activities of the brain. Memories are produced and preserved in particular parts of the brain, and they are consolidated overtime via the development of neuronal connections. When we remember a memory, certain neurons are stimulated, helping us to recollect the information. The process of memory development and recall is assumed to be impacted by a variety of elements, including experience, emotion, and attention.

Another key function of the brain is to govern movement. The brain organizes and regulates our motions via the creation of electrical impulses that are communicated to our muscles, enabling us to accomplish complicated tasks such as typing on a keyboard or playing a musical instrument. This process is regulated by certain parts of the brain, including the motor cortex, which is responsible for the planning and execution of movement, and the cerebellum, which coordinates and fine-tunes our motions.

The brain also plays a key role in controlling our ideas, emotions, and actions. This process is carried out by certain parts of the brain, including the prefrontal cortex, which is responsible for decision-making, and the amygdala, which is responsible for regulating emotions. Our ideas, emotions, and actions are impacted by a variety of variables, including experience, heredity, and hormones, and they may be changed via therapy, medicine, and other treatments.

Finally, the brain is responsible for consciousness, which is our subjective perception of the world around us.

Consciousness is assumed to be a product of the intricate connections between various parts of the brain, and it is thought to entail the integration of sensory information, memory, and cognition. Consciousness is still not completely understood, but scientists are making progress in understanding the basic systems and how they contribute to our view of the world.

In conclusion, the brain is an extraordinarily complex and sophisticated organ that plays a key role in managing our ideas, emotions, actions, movements, and awareness. Despite its complexity, scientists have been able to make enormous progress in understanding how the brain functions and this knowledge is helping to develop novel therapies for brain illnesses and to boost our capacity to learn, think, and create. Further study into the brain and its activities will continue to reveal insights into how it operates and how we may utilize this knowledge to enhance our lives.

The human brain is a fascinating and complicated organ that is responsible for a vast variety of processes, including sensation, perception, movement, emotion, thinking, and consciousness. Understanding the functioning of the brain involves a multidisciplinary approach, pulling from domains such as anatomy, physiology, psychology, and neuroscience.

One of the main properties of the brain is its capacity to adapt and change in response to new experiences, a process known as neuroplasticity. This implies that the brain may rewire itself, generating new connections and pathways between neurons, in response to new experiences, learning, and damage. This capacity to modify and adapt is what enables us to acquire new skills, heal from injuries, and overcome constraints.

Another essential element of the brain is its specialization. Different parts of the brain are specialized to execute certain activities, such as processing visual information, regulating movement, or managing emotions. For example, the visual cortex is specialized for processing visual information, whereas the motor cortex is specialized for directing movement. This specialization helps the brain to effectively digest enormous volumes of information and react appropriately to varied circumstances.

The brain also has a hierarchical structure, with higher-level areas processing information from lower-level regions. This implies that information from the senses, such as sight, hearing, and touch, is initially processed in lower-level areas before being transferred to higher-level regions for further processing. This permits us to make sense of the world around us and behave accordingly.

One of the most impressive features of the brain is its capacity to retain and recover memories. Memories are stored in particular areas of the brain, and the process of recall requires the activation of specific neuronal circuits that relate to the memory. This process is regulated by a variety of variables, including the strength of the synaptic connections between neurons, the degree of attention devoted to the event, and the emotional state of the person at the time of the encounter.

The brain also plays a key role in controlling our emotions and behavior. Emotions and actions are governed by certain parts of the brain, including the amygdala, which is involved in the processing of emotions, and the prefrontal cortex, which is involved in decision-making and impulse control. Hormonal and genetic variables also have a role in controlling emotions and actions.

Finally, the brain is also responsible for forming our subjective perception of the world, known as consciousness. Consciousness is assumed to develop from the intricate connections between various parts of the brain, and scientists are currently attempting to understand the fundamental principles of this intriguing phenomenon.

The human brain is an immensely complex and sophisticated organ that is responsible for a vast variety of processes, including sensation, perception, movement, emotion, thinking, and awareness. Understanding the functioning of the brain takes a multidisciplinary approach, pulling from domains such as anatomy, physiology, psychology, and neuroscience, and will continue to bring insights into how we may better our lives.

The brain is an extraordinarily complicated organ, and understanding how it works may be a struggle. Here are some of the essential stages involved in the functioning of the brain:

Sensory processing: The first stage in how the brain operates is sensory processing. The brain takes information from the senses, such as sight, hearing, touch, taste, and smell, and processes this information in specific parts of the brain. This information is then passed to higher-level areas for further processing.

Perception: Once the information from the senses has been processed, the brain utilizes this information to generate perceptions of the world around us. Perception is the process by which the brain makes sense of the information it receives from the senses and combines this information into a cohesive image of the environment.

Attention: Attention is a vital feature of perception and is necessary for the proper processing of information. Attention permits us to selectively concentrate on some parts of our surroundings and disregard others, depending on what is most essential or relevant in a particular moment.

Movement: Movement is governed by specific parts of the brain, including the motor cortex and the basal ganglia. These areas operate together to coordinate the muscles and limbs to create movement.

Emotion: Emotions are governed by specific parts of the brain, including the amygdala, hypothalamus, and prefrontal cortex. These areas operate together to form our emotional experiences and impact our behavior.

Memory: The brain stores and retrieves memories in particular locations, and the process of recall requires the activation of specific neural pathways that match the memory. This process is regulated by a variety of variables, including the strength of the synaptic connections between neurons, the degree of attention devoted to the event, and the emotional state of the person at the time of the encounter.

Decision-making: Decision-making is governed by the prefrontal cortex, which is engaged in impulse control and executive function. This part of the brain collaborates with other regions to help us make choices, plan activities, and manage our behavior.

Consciousness: Consciousness is assumed to originate from the intricate connections between various parts of the brain, and scientists are currently attempting to understand the fundamental mechanics of this phenomenon. Consciousness enables us to perceive the world and reflect on our experiences and is a unique and extraordinary character of the human brain.

These stages give a simplified overview of how the brain works, although many of the processes involved are significantly more complicated and include the interaction of numerous areas of the brain. Despite the complexity of the brain, scientists are making progress in understanding its functioning, and this knowledge is enabling us to enhance our lives in several ways.

The Different Parts of the Brain

The human brain is a highly integrated, complex system made up of a variety of specialized components that cooperate to control our body's and mind's functions. To comprehend how the brain functions and the significance of preserving brain health, one must have a thorough awareness of the many areas of the brain and their respective roles.

We'll talk about some of the important brain structures and their functions in this conversation.

The cerebral cortex, which is the brain's outer layer, is in charge of several crucial processes like perception, movement, attention, and conscious cognition. The frontal lobe, parietal lobe, temporal lobe, and occipital lobe are the four major divisions of the cerebral cortex. Each of these areas is in charge of particular tasks like processing sensory data, managing movement, and controlling voice.

The frontal lobe is the largest of the four major parts of the cerebral cortex and is in charge of several crucial processes, such as decision-making, problem-solving, and movement regulation. Our emotions and social behavior are also controlled by the frontal lobe.

The processing of sensory information, such as touch, temperature, and pain, is done by the parietal lobe. Additionally, this lobe is involved in the integration of sensory data, spatial awareness, and mathematical processing.

The processing of auditory information is carried out by the temporal lobe, which is also involved in memory, speech, and language. The temporal lobe also plays a role in controlling emotions and time perception.

The Occipital Lobe: Situated near the back of the brain, the occipital lobe is in charge of processing visual information. This lobe is essential for our capacity to perceive, analyze, and comprehend visual data.

The creation and recall of memories are controlled by the hippocampus, a small but significant portion of the brain. Our capacity to learn and remember new knowledge as well as spatial navigation depends on this area of the brain.

The basal ganglia are a collection of nuclei that play a role in controlling movement and coordination. This area of the brain is crucial for our capacity to carry out complicated movements and is also involved in the learning of new movements.

The Thalamus: The Thalamus is a sizable, almond-shaped brain structure that is in charge of sending sensory data to the cerebral cortex. It is situated in the center of the brain. Our capacity to receive and integrate sensory data, such as that from touch, vision, and hearing, depends on this area of the brain.

The portion of the brain that links the spinal cord to the rest of the brain is known as the brainstem. This area of the brain is in charge of managing vital life-sustaining processes including breathing and heart rate as well as our sleep-wake cycle.

The base of the brainstem is home to the cerebellum, a tiny but significant portion of the brain. Movement, balance, and coordination are coordinated by this area of the brain. The cerebellum also plays a role in controlling speech and fine motor skills.

In conclusion, the human brain is a sophisticated and intricately connected system made up of a variety of specialized structures that cooperate to control our mental and physical functions. Understanding the roles of the many brain regions is crucial to comprehend how the brain functions and the significance of sustaining brain health.

Communication in the Brain: Its Importance

Neurons in the brain communicate with one another through a process called neural signaling, commonly referred to as brain communication. Many different processes, including perception, movement, emotion, memory, decision-making, and awareness, depend on this mechanism. Understanding the significance of brain communication might enhance our appreciation of the brain's complexity and the amazing ways in which it enables us to interact with our environment.

Here are some of the critical phases in brain communication and why they are so crucial:

The initial stage of brain communication is the signal's start, which is brought on by modifications to a neuron's electrical or chemical makeup. Numerous events, such as the receipt of a sensory signal, the release of a neurotransmitter, or the activation of a particular neuronal route, might result in this alteration.

Once a signal has been initiated, it is transferred down the length of the neuron, from the dendrites to the cell body, and finally to the terminal boutons, traveling along the axon. The arrival of the signal to the terminal boutons causes the release of neurotransmitters. The signal is carried via the movement of charged particles, such as ions.

Release of neurotransmitters: Chemicals known as neurotransmitters are released by one neuron's terminal boutons and bind to particular receptors on the dendrites of another neuron. This binding causes the receiving neuron's electrical or chemical characteristics to alter, enabling the signal to go to another part of the brain.

Receptor activation: The transmission of the signal depends on the activation of receptors on the receiving neuron. Different neurotransmitters attach to various receptor types and depending on which receptor is triggered, the receiving cell will respond in a particular way. This makes it possible for the brain to have an advanced and complicated communication system.

Signal integration: The signal is incorporated into the activity of the receiving neuron after it has been passed from one neuron to another. The number of neurotransmitters released, the quality of the synaptic connections between the neurons, and the existence of concurrently conveyed signals are only a few of the variables that have an impact on this integration.

Feedback mechanisms: Feedback mechanisms are essential for controlling brain activity and making sure the system works properly. For instance, other signals, such as hormones or other substances, can affect the release of neurotransmitters, and repeated activation can alter the strength of neuronal connections.

The receiving neuron's output, which can result in further signal transmission, the activation of muscles or glands, or the creation of conscious experience, is the last stage of brain communication. The sort of signal that was received, the kind of receptor that was triggered, and the particular neurological pathways involved all affect the receiving neuron's output.

Brain communication is significant because it enables the quick and effective transfer of information throughout the brain, enabling us to connect with our environment and carry out a variety of tasks. Many of the processes that we take for granted, like seeing, hearing, moving, feeling, and thinking, would not be possible without efficient brain communication.

In addition, the sophisticated network of neuronal transmission underlies the brain's plasticity, or capacity to adapt to experience. Learning and adapting are made possible by the brain's capacity for change in response to experience, which is an essential aspect of brain health and well-being.

In conclusion, brain communication is a complicated and sophisticated process that is crucial

The intricacy of brain communication and its relevance to our general well-being cannot be emphasized. In this part, we will go further into the stages involved in brain communication to better grasp its relevance.

Synaptic plasticity: One of the most fundamental characteristics of brain communication is the capacity of synapses, or the connections between neurons, to alter in response to experience. This mechanism, known as synaptic plasticity, enables the brain to adapt and adjust its communication channels depending on new knowledge or experiences. For example, frequent exposure to a specific stimulus might lead to the strengthening of the connections between neurons, allowing for quicker and more efficient transmission of messages.

Neural networks: The connection between neurons produces sophisticated networks of information inside the brain. These networks are responsible for a vast variety of processes, including perception, emotion, memory, decision-making, and awareness. The activity of these networks is dynamic, with various areas of the brain working together to complete certain tasks. Understanding the functioning of these networks is crucial for understanding how the brain operates and the significance of brain communication.

Cognitive functions: Brain communication is crucial for the functioning of the cognitive processes that allow us to think, reason, and solve problems. For example, the connection between neurons in the frontal cortex and other parts of the brain is critical for decision-making, planning, and executive processes. Similarly, the connection between neurons in the hippocampus and other locations is crucial for the creation and recall of memories.

Emotional regulation: Brain communication also plays a vital function in managing our emotions. The connection between the amygdala and other parts of the brain is critical for the processing of emotional information, including the perception of danger and the management of fear and anxiety. Additionally, the connection between the prefrontal cortex and other areas is crucial for the regulation of emotional reactions, enabling us to manage our emotions and respond properly to diverse circumstances.

Sensory processing: The connection between neurons is also crucial for the processing of sensory information. For example, the connection between neurons in the visual cortex and other areas is required for the sense of sight, whereas the communication between neurons in the auditory cortex and other regions is crucial for the experience of sound. The fast and efficient transmission of sensory information enables us to react swiftly and effectively to the environment around us.

Motor control: Brain connection is also crucial for the control of movement. The connection between neurons in the motor cortex and other areas is crucial for the planning and execution of movements, while the communication between neurons in the spinal cord and other regions is critical for the regulation of reflexes and automatic movements. The fast and accurate communication between these areas helps us to move with accuracy and elegance.

Learning and memory: Brain communication plays a vital part in the processes of learning and remembering. For example, the communication between neurons in the hippocampus and other areas is required for the creation of long-term memories, whereas the connection between neurons in the cortex and other regions is crucial for the recall of memories. Additionally, the connection between neurons in the basal ganglia and other locations is crucial for the establishment of habits and the control of repeated actions.

Consciousness:Finally,brain communication is important for the production of conscious experience. The connection between neurons in the thalamus and other areas is required for the integration of sensory information, whereas the communication between neurons in the cortex and other regions is crucial for the creation of ideas, emotions, and other elements of conscious experience. The complicated network of communication between neurons enables us to perceive the environment in a rich and complex manner.

In conclusion, the significance of brain communication cannot be emphasized. It is the basis upon which all of our perceptions, actions, emotions, memories, choices.

Enhancing Brain Function

Enhancing brain function is a key element of sustaining excellent mental health and general well-being. There is a range of strategies to increase brain function, ranging from lifestyle modifications to particular workouts and hobbies. In this part, we will discuss some of the most effective strategies for increasing brain function.

Exercise: Regular physical exercise is one of the greatest strategies to increase brain function. Exercise has been demonstrated to improve cognitive performance, increase brain volume, and accelerate the creation of new neurons in the brain. Exercise also boosts the synthesis of neurotransmitters, such as dopamine and serotonin, which are vital for mood control and motivation.

Sleep: Getting adequate quality sleep is also vital for increasing brain function. Sleep is vital for the consolidation of memories and the processing of information. Additionally, sleep deprivation has been associated with a range of cognitive deficits, including lower attention, memory impairment, and poor executive function.

Nutrition: A healthy diet is crucial for brain function. Consuming a diet that is rich in fruits, vegetables, whole grains, and healthy fats may assist to preserve cognitive function and lower the risk of age-related cognitive decline. Additionally, studies have indicated that some foods, such as blueberries, salmon, and walnuts, may increase brain function by delivering vital nutrients for brain health.

Mental stimulation: Challenging the brain with mental stimulation is also vital for boosting brain function. This may include activities such as reading, learning a new skill, or playing mental games. Mental stimulation helps to sustain cognitive function and may also increase memory and attention.

Stress management: Chronic stress has been related to a range of deleterious impacts on brain function, including impaired memory and concentration, and increased anxiety and depression. To boost brain function, it is vital to acquire appropriate stress management practices, such as mindfulness meditation, yoga, or exercise.

Social contact: Social interaction has been demonstrated to be vital for brain function, as it may promote cognitive performance, increase the synthesis of neurotransmitters, and lessen the risk of sadness and anxiety. Spending time with friends and family, volunteering, or joining a social group may all assist to increase brain function.

Brain training programs: There are also a variety of brain training programs and apps available that are aimed to boost brain function. These programs often contain activities such as memory games, focus challenges, and problem-solving exercises. While the efficacy of these programs is currently the topic of continuing study, many individuals find them useful for preserving cognitive function and boosting brain function.

Meditation: Meditation has been demonstrated to provide a multitude of advantages for brain function, including greater attention, better memory, and decreased stress and anxiety. Regular practice of meditation may assist to increase brain function by enhancing the capacity to concentrate and by eliminating distractions.

Music: Listening to music has also been demonstrated to have favorable impacts on brain function. Music has been demonstrated to increase memory, decrease stress, and promote mood. Additionally, playing a musical instrument has been demonstrated to increase cognitive performance, since it demands coordination, attention, and memory.

In conclusion, there are various techniques to boost brain function. By adopting a mix of these tactics into your everyday life, you may assist to preserve cognitive performance and enhance overall brain health. Additionally, it is crucial to obtain the counsel of a healthcare practitioner before commencing any new activities or treatments to verify that they are safe and suitable for you.

One technique to increase brain function is through participating in physical activity. Exercise has been found to stimulate the synthesis of neurochemicals in the brain, such as dopamine and serotonin, which have a role in mood regulation and motivation. Additionally, regular physical exercise has been found to improve cognitive performance, expand brain volume, and accelerate the creation of new neurons in the brain. Exercise may also assist to alleviate stress and anxiety, which can have harmful impacts on brain function.

Another strategy to increase brain function is by obtaining adequate quality sleep. Sleep is necessary for the consolidation of memories and the processing of information. Chronic sleep deprivation has been associated with a range of cognitive deficits, such as reduced attention, memory impairment, and poor executive function. To boost brain performance, it is necessary to obtain adequate sleep and keep a regular sleep routine.

Nutrition is also a key part of enhancing brain function. Consuming a diet that is rich in fruits, vegetables, whole grains, and healthy fats may assist to preserve cognitive function and lower the risk of age-related cognitive decline. Additionally, some foods, such as blueberries, salmon, and walnuts, may increase brain function by delivering critical nutrients for brain health. It is also vital to avoid eating a diet that is heavy in processed foods, sugar, and saturated fats since these foods have been related to harmful impacts on brain function.

Mental stimulation is also vital for boosting brain function. This may include activities such as reading, learning a new skill, or playing mental games. Mental stimulation helps to sustain cognitive function and may also increase memory and attention. Additionally, participating in mental stimulation may assist to alleviate stress and anxiety, which can have harmful impacts on brain function.

Stress management is another crucial part of boosting brain function. Chronic stress has been related to a range of deleterious impacts on brain function, including impaired memory and concentration, and increased anxiety and depression. To boost brain function, it is vital to create an appropriate stress management

Staying Mentally Active

Staying intellectually engaged is a vital component of sustaining cognitive function and general brain health. The brain is a sophisticated and adaptable organ, and participating in activities that challenge the intellect may assist to preserve cognitive function, lower the risk of age-related cognitive decline, and boost general brain health. In this post, we will cover numerous ways for remaining intellectually active and the advantages of mental stimulation.

Engage in Challenging Activities: Engaging in activities that challenge the mind, such as solving puzzles, learning a new skill, or playing brain games, is one of the most effective methods to keep intellectually active. These exercises may assist to enhance attention, memory, and executive function, and can also minimize the risk of age-related cognitive decline.

Learn a New Language: Learning a new language may be a tough and rewarding way to keep cognitively busy. Not only does it test the brain, but it also introduces you to various cultures and viewpoints, and may boost memory and concentration.

Read Regularly: Reading is an excellent method to keep intellectually active since it exposes the brain to fresh knowledge and ideas. Whether you enjoy fiction, non-fiction, or a mix of both, reading may help to preserve cognitive function, minimize the risk of age-related cognitive decline, and enhance memory and attention.

Engage in Social Activities: Engaging in social activities, such as spending time with friends and family, volunteering, or joining a group, is another fantastic way to keep intellectually active. These exercises may assist to decrease stress and anxiety, which can have harmful impacts on brain function and can also enhance memory and concentration.

Stay Physically Active: Regular physical activity is not only necessary for physical health, but it is also crucial for mental health. Exercise has been found to stimulate the synthesis of neurochemicals in the brain, such as dopamine and serotonin, which have a role in mood regulation and motivation. Additionally, regular physical exercise has been found to improve cognitive performance, expand brain volume, and accelerate the creation of new neurons in the brain.

Get Enough Sleep: Sleep is crucial for the consolidation of memories and the processing of information. Chronic sleep deprivation has been associated with a range of cognitive deficits, such as reduced attention, memory impairment, and poor executive function. To boost brain performance, it is necessary to obtain adequate sleep and keep a regular sleep routine.

Consume a Healthy Diet: Consuming a diet that is rich in fruits, vegetables, whole grains, and healthy fats will assist to preserve cognitive function and lower the risk of age-related cognitive decline.

Additionally, some foods, such as blueberries, salmon, and walnuts, may increase brain function by delivering critical nutrients for brain health. It is also vital to avoid eating a diet that is heavy in processed foods, sugar, and saturated fats since these foods have been related to harmful impacts on brain function.

Manage Stress: Chronic stress has been related to a range of harmful impacts on brain function, including impaired memory and concentration, and increased anxiety and depression. To boost brain function, it is vital to adopt appropriate stress management practices, such as exercise, meditation, or counseling.

In conclusion, remaining intellectually active is a vital component of sustaining cognitive function and general brain health. Whether you like participating in demanding activities, learning a new language, reading frequently, engaging in social events, remaining physically active, getting enough sleep, eating a good diet, or managing stress, there are many different techniques for staying intellectually engaged. By implementing these tactics into your daily routine, you may boost brain function, lower the risk of age-related cognitive decline, and retain cognitive performance long into the old life.

Brain Training

Brain training is a strategy for enhancing cognitive performance via participating in activities and exercises meant to challenge the brain. The notion of brain training is founded on the idea of neuroplasticity, which refers to the brain's capacity to alter and adapt in response to experience. The purpose of brain training is to promote cognitive function and improve mental performance by strengthening the connections between neurons in the brain.

There are many various forms of brain training activities, including cognitive training exercises, memory training games, and mindfulness techniques. Cognitive training activities often concentrate on boosting attention, memory, and executive function, whereas memory training games are aimed to increase memory abilities. Mindfulness techniques, such as meditation and yoga, are intended to relieve stress and anxiety, This may have detrimental repercussions on cognitive function.

The benefits of brain training are extensively known, and research has demonstrated that brain training may boost cognitive performance, lessen the risk of age-related cognitive decline, and promote overall brain health. In addition to these benefits, brain training has also been found to boost mood and diminish feelings of sadness and worry.

One of the primary advantages of brain training is the enhancement of attention and executive function. Attention and executive function are key abilities that are required for everyday tasks, such as working, driving, and managing funds. By participating in activities that test attention and executive function, the brain may build up its capacity to concentrate and prioritize tasks.

Memory is another cognitive skill that may be enhanced via brain training. Memory training games and activities may assist to strengthen memory recall, as well as boost the speed and accuracy of memory retrieval. Additionally, memory training has been found to increase working memory, which is crucial for keeping and processing information in real time.

Mindfulness techniques, such as meditation and yoga, are also significant components of brain training. These activities may assist to decrease stress and anxiety, which can have harmful consequences on cognitive performance. Additionally, mindfulness activities have been demonstrated to increase attention, working memory, and executive function.

In conclusion, brain training is a powerful technique for increasing cognitive performance, minimizing the risk of age-related cognitive decline, and promoting general brain health. Whether you prefer cognitive training activities, memory training games, or mindfulness techniques, there are many different methods to participate in brain training. By adding brain training into your everyday routine, you may preserve cognitive function, increase mental performance, and lower the risk of age-related cognitive decline.

Conclusion

The Importance of Maintaining Brain Health

In conclusion, preserving brain health is vital for general wellness and meaningful life. The brain is a complicated organ that plays a key role in controlling emotions, thoughts, and behavior. As we age, the brain might become less efficient and cognitive decline can occur, which can significantly affect everyday living. However, there are activities that may be performed to preserve brain health and slow down the aging process of the brain.

First and foremost, a healthy lifestyle is vital for preserving brain health. Eating a balanced diet that is rich in fruits, vegetables, whole grains, and healthy fats may give the brain the nutrients it needs to operate effectively. Regular exercise has also been demonstrated to promote brain function and improve memory and cognitive performance.

In addition, remaining intellectually engaged is a vital aspect of preserving brain health. Engaging in activities that engage the brain, such as reading, playing games, and solving puzzles may assist to preserve cognitive function and lower the risk of age-related cognitive decline. Brain training activities, such as cognitive training exercises and memory training games, may also aid to improve cognitive performance and promote general brain health.

Finally, decreasing stress and cultivating mindfulness are crucial components of preserving brain health. Chronic stress has been found to have deleterious effects on cognitive performance and raise the chance of age-related cognitive decline. By adopting mindfulness techniques, such as meditation and yoga, into your routine, you may decrease stress and increase brain function.

In conclusion, preserving brain health is vital for a great existence. By living a healthy lifestyle, participating in cognitively challenging activities, and decreasing stress, you may preserve brain health and lower the risk of age-related cognitive decline. By taking care of your brain, you can guarantee that you have the cognitive function and mental performance you need to live life to the fullest

In addition to the actions indicated in the preceding conclusion, there are a few additional steps that may be followed to preserve brain health and slow down the aging process of the brain.

One such step is obtaining proper sleep. Sleep is crucial for the brain to operate correctly since it is during sleep that the brain analyzes and consolidates memories, repairs damage, and eliminates waste. Aim for 7-9 hours of quality sleep each night to preserve brain health.

Another stage is to push your brain by acquiring new skills and hobbies. This might involve learning a new language, pursuing a new pastime, or taking on additional duties at work. By regularly pushing the brain, you may establish new neural connections and strengthen old ones, which can assist to preserve brain health.

Social involvement is also a crucial component of preserving brain function. Studies have indicated that social involvement and social support may enhance cognitive performance and lower the risk of age-related cognitive decline. Engage in activities that enable you to engage with people, such as volunteering, joining clubs or groups, or just spending time with friends and family.

In addition, avoiding exposure to harmful chemicals, such as cigarettes, alcohol, and narcotics, is vital for preserving brain health. These drugs may harm brain cells and significantly influence cognitive function. By avoiding these chemicals, you may safeguard your brain and lower the risk of age-related cognitive decline.

Finally, decreasing stress is a vital aspect of preserving brain health. Chronic stress has been found to have deleterious effects on cognitive performance and raise the chance of age-related cognitive decline. Engage in activities that assist to alleviate stress, such as mindfulness techniques, exercise, and spending time in nature.

In conclusion, preserving brain health is vital for a great existence. By living a healthy lifestyle, participating in cognitively stimulating activities, decreasing stress, and pushing your brain with new skills and experiences, you may preserve brain health and lower the risk of age-related cognitive decline. By taking care of your brain, you can guarantee that you have the cognitive function and mental performance you need to live life to the fullest.

Summary of important Points

The significance of preserving brain health cannot be emphasized. The brain is the control center of the body and plays a critical role in controlling emotions, ideas, and behavior. With aging, the brain may become less efficient, and cognitive decline can develop, which can significantly affect everyday living. However, there are activities that may be performed to preserve brain health and slow down the aging process of the brain.

One of the major components of sustaining brain health is having a healthy lifestyle. Eating a balanced diet that is rich in fruits, vegetables, whole grains, and healthy fats may give the brain the nutrients it needs to operate effectively. Regular exercise has also been demonstrated to promote brain function and improve memory and cognitive performance.

Staying intellectually busy is another crucial part of preserving brain health. Engaging in activities that engage the brain, such as reading, playing games, and solving puzzles may assist to preserve cognitive function and lower the risk of age-related cognitive decline. Challenging the brain with new skills and experiences, such as learning a new language or taking up a new hobby, may also assist to form new neural connections and reinforce old ones.

Adequate sleep is also vital for sustaining brain function. Sleep is crucial for the brain to operate correctly since it is during sleep that the brain analyzes and consolidates memories, repairs damage, and eliminates waste. Aim for 7-9 hours of quality sleep each night to preserve brain health.

Social involvement is also a crucial component of preserving brain function. Studies have indicated that social involvement and social support may enhance cognitive performance and lower the risk of age-related cognitive decline. Engage in activities that enable you to engage with people, such as volunteering, joining clubs or groups, or just spending time with friends and family.

Reducing exposure to harmful chemicals, such as cigarettes, alcohol, and narcotics is vital for sustaining brain health. These drugs may harm brain cells and significantly influence cognitive function. By avoiding these chemicals, you may safeguard your brain and lower the risk of age-related cognitive decline.

Finally, decreasing stress is a vital aspect of preserving brain health. Chronic stress has been found to have deleterious effects on cognitive performance and raise the chance of age-related cognitive decline. Engage in activities that assist to alleviate stress, such as mindfulness techniques, exercise, and spending time in nature.

In conclusion, preserving brain health is vital for a great existence. By living a healthy lifestyle, participating in cognitively stimulating activities, decreasing stress, and pushing your brain with new skills and experiences, you may preserve brain health and lower the risk of age-related cognitive decline. By taking care of your brain, you can guarantee that you have the cognitive function and mental performance you need to live life to the fullest.

Summary of Key Points in Maintaining Brain Health

1. Lead a healthy lifestyle:\sEat a balanced diet that is rich in fruits, vegetables, whole grains, and healthy fats

2. Engage in frequent physical activity

3. Stay intellectually active:\sEngage in activities that engage the brain, such as reading, playing games, and solving problems

4. Challenge the brain with new abilities and experiences, such as learning a new language or taking up a new activity

5. Get proper sleep:

Aim for 7-9 hours of decent sleep each night

6. Foster social engagement:\sEngage in activities that enable you to connect with people, such as volunteering, joining clubs or organizations, or spending time with friends and family

7. Avoid harmful substances:

Reduce exposure to hazardous chemicals, such as cigarettes, alcohol, and drugs

8. Reduce stress:\sEngage in activities that assist to reduce stress, such as mindfulness techniques, exercise, and spending time in nature

By following these procedures, you may preserve brain health and lower the risk of age-related cognitive decline. By taking care of your brain, you can guarantee that you have the cognitive function and mental performance you need to live life to the fullest.

Final Thoughts

Final Thoughts on the Importance of Maintaining Brain Health:

Maintaining brain health is a vital part of overall health and well-being. Our brains play a significant part in all areas of our lives, from our capacity to comprehend and absorb information, to our emotions and conduct, to our relationships and personal life. The human brain is a complex and sophisticated organ that has the potential to evolve and adapt throughout our lives, which makes it necessary to preserve its health and function.

The key to sustaining brain health rests in adopting favorable lifestyle choices and participating in activities that enhance cognitive well-being. This involves adopting a healthy lifestyle, remaining cognitively engaged, obtaining appropriate sleep, developing social involvement, avoiding hazardous drugs, and lowering stress. By participating in these activities, you may lower the risk of age-related cognitive decline, improve cognitive performance, and increase your overall quality of life.

In today's fast-paced society, it may be tempting to disregard our mental and physical health. However, spending the time to concentrate on preserving brain health is a worthy investment. By taking care of your brain, you can guarantee that you have the cognitive function and mental performance you need to excel in all parts of your life.

It's never too late to start taking care of your brain. Whether you're young or elderly, there are basic activities you can take to preserve brain health. Whether you want to engage in physical exercise, participate in social activities, or engage in cerebral stimulation, there are numerous strategies to promote brain function and improve overall health.

In conclusion, preserving brain health is a vital part of total well-being.

By participating in activities that promote cognitive wellness, minimizing stress, avoiding hazardous drugs, and adopting good lifestyle choices, you may guarantee that your brain stays healthy and working at its best. So, take the time to concentrate on your brain health, and enjoy all the advantages that come with a healthy, functioning brain.

- Recognize the significance of brain health:

Acknowledge the essential role that the brain plays in our overall health and well-being understand that preserving brain health is vital for success and pleasure in life.

- Make good lifestyle choices:

Lead a healthy lifestyle by eating a balanced diet, participating in regular physical exercise, and obtaining appropriate sleep.

Foster social connection and decrease stress by engaging in activities that enable you to communicate with people and participate in activities that promote relaxation

Avoid harmful substances such as alcohol, drugs, and tobacco

- Stay mentally active:

Engage in activities that engage the brain, such as reading, playing games, and solving problems

Challenge the brain with new abilities and experiences, such as learning a new language or taking up a new activity.

- Exercise regularly:

Physical exercise is vital for brain health and may enhance cognitive function and minimize the risk of age-related cognitive decline.

- Get sufficient sleep:

Aim for 7-9 hours of adequate sleep each night to promote healthy brain function.

- Foster social engagement:

Engage in activities that enable you to engage with people, such as volunteering, joining clubs or groups, or spending time with friends and family.

- Reduce stress:

Engage in activities that assist to relieve stress, such as mindfulness techniques, exercise, and spending time in nature.

- Encourage continual learning:

Keep the brain active and engaged by continuing to learn new things, whether it be by attending courses, reading, or participating in other intellectually challenging activities.

By following these procedures, you may preserve brain health and lower the risk of age-related cognitive decline. Additionally, taking care of your brain may enhance your overall quality of life and raise your chances of success and happiness in all parts of your life. Whether you're young or elderly, it's never too late to start taking care of your brain. By adopting good lifestyle choices and participating in activities that promote cognitive wellness, you can guarantee that your brain stays healthy and works at its best.

www.ingramcontent.com/pod-product-compliance
Lightning Source LLC
Chambersburg PA
CBHW071140220526
45467CB00015B/1610